The healings of (psilocybin)magic mushroom for beginners

Exploring the Impact of Magic Mushrooms on Mental Health

Maggret Erik

Chapter One...3

Exploring the Impact of Magic Mushrooms on Mental Health 3

Chapter Two 15

Research on psilocybin's medicinal effects has evolved 15

Chapter Three 22

Magic mushroom usage in traditional cultures 22

Chapter Four 28

How psilocybin is converted by the body to psilocin 28

Chapter Five 39

Important discoveries made during clinical trials regarding mental health issues...........39

Chapter Six 51

Summary of research on depression diseases 51

Chapter Seven 71

Things to Think About:.................................71

Chapter One

Exploring the Impact of Magic Mushrooms on Mental Health

Introduction

Magic mushrooms, known for their psychedelic properties induced by the presence of the compound psilocybin, have captivated human curiosity and cultural practices for centuries. In recent years, a burgeoning wave of scientific interest has propelled psilocybin into the spotlight as a potential therapeutic agent for mental health conditions. This exploration delves into the intricate relationship between psilocybin, derived from magic mushrooms, and its impact on mental well-being. As societal attitudes shift, so does the attention toward the therapeutic potential of these naturally occurring substances. This study aims to unravel the historical context, dissect recent research findings, and contemplate the future implications of harnessing the therapeutic potential of psilocybin in the realm of mental health. By navigating this multifaceted landscape, we seek to shed light on the promise and challenges associated with integrating magic mushrooms into contemporary mental health treatments.

Definition of Magic Mushrooms and Psilocybin

Psilocybin is a hallucinogenic substance that is naturally present in some kinds of mushrooms, most notably those that are in the Psilocybe genus. Psilocybin is a hallucinogenic drug that alters consciousness and influences mood, perception, and cognition. Psilocybin is transformed by the body into its active form, psilocin, which combines with serotonin receptors in the brain to produce psychedelic effects.

Psilocybin- and/or psilocin- containing mushrooms are known

as magic mushrooms or psychedelic mushrooms. These mushrooms have long been employed in a variety of traditional and religious rituals, especially by native cultures in places like Mesoamerica. The term "magic mushrooms" refers to a general word that includes a variety of hallucinogenic species. Taking magic mushrooms can cause intense hallucinations, changes in temporal perception, and deep spiritual experiences. Magic mushrooms and psilocybin have both attracted attention recently due to possible therapeutic uses in mental health studies.

Growing interest in psilocybin's potential as a therapy

A paradigm change in the study and practice of mental health is being brought about by the increased interest in psilocybin's therapeutic potential. Magic mushrooms, which contain the hallucinogenic substance psilocybin and have historically been linked to counterculture movements and recreational use, have drawn the interest of researchers, medical professionals, and members of the general public in recent times.

The growing interest in the therapeutic potential of psilocybin is due to a number of factors. First, there is evidence from a number of convincing early investigations and clinical trials that psilocybin may have special advantages for a range of mental health issues. Its potential effectiveness in reducing symptoms of anxiety, sadness, and post-traumatic stress disorder (PTSD) is being studied by researchers.

Moreover, the constraints associated with traditional mental health drugs have prompted the investigation of novel and alternative methods. With its unique brain effects, psilocybin offers a new therapy option for mental health conditions that don't respond to standard therapies. Psilocybin-induced psychedelic experiences are thought to cause significant changes in consciousness, which may provide users with fresh viewpoints and life lessons.

Interest in psilocybin has also been greatly aided by the change in public perceptions of psychedelics. There is a growing willingness to investigate the therapeutic potential of psychedelic substances in a monitored and regulated medical setting as public attitudes about them change and the stigmas associated with them fade.

The growing interest in psilocybin's therapeutic uses represents a shift from conventional methods of treating mental illness as research into the drug's complex brain effects and mechanisms continues. Not only is the study of psilocybin's therapeutic potential scientific, but it also reflects a broader cultural reevaluation of the possible benefits of psychedelics for improving mental health. This increasing attention opens the door to a greater comprehension of the potential substantial effects on mental health therapy that psilocybin and magic mushrooms may have in the future.

The investigation's goal is to comprehend the effects on mental wellness.

The aim of investigating psilocybin's effects on mental health stems from the realization that it has transformative potential that goes beyond traditional psychiatric therapies. This investigation aims to clarify the intricate relationship between psilocybin and mental health, with a particular emphasis on three main goals:

1. Discover Therapeutic Potential: The main goal is to investigate the growing corpus of evidence that indicates psilocybin may be therapeutically beneficial for those dealing with mental health issues. This investigation seeks to illuminate the subtleties of psilocybin's brain interactions in order to provide light on the drug's potential for reducing PTSD, anxiety, and depressive symptoms.

2. Contextualize Historical Practices: The investigation aims to provide historical background on the various civilizations' historical applications of magic mushrooms. It attempts to give a thorough background to the current resurgence of interest in psilocybin by looking at customs and societal attitudes around psychedelics. This historical perspective sheds light on the cultural, spiritual, and medicinal aspects of magic mushrooms that have been connected to them throughout human history.

3. Handle Ethical and Practical Issues: This investigation recognizes the ethical issues related to the use of psychedelics in mental health treatment, going beyond the realm of science. It aims to negotiate the difficulties involved in guaranteeing the security, legitimacy, and responsible use of psilocybin. The goal is to contribute to a responsible and educated discourse on the possible integration of psilocybin into standard mental health care by addressing ethical problems and practical considerations.

Chapter Two

Research on psilocybin's medicinal effects has evolved

The development of psilocybin research from a topic of speculative interest to a rapidly expanding area of scientific study is a fascinating trip. This development is divided into discrete stages, each of which adds to our comprehension of the compound's possible medical uses:

1. Initial Research and Cultural Origins:

- Throughout the 20th century, countercultural movements drove the investigation of psychedelic chemicals, which frequently overlapped with early studies

• Early research, including that of Richard Alpert (later Ram Dass) and Timothy Leary, established the groundwork for our knowledge of the subjective experiences that psilocybin induces.

2. Failures and Regulatory Obstacles:

• In the late 1960s and early 1970s, regulatory agencies placed limitations on their research because of worries about psychedelic use for recreational purposes.

- The scientific investigation of psilocybin was restricted throughout this prohibitionary period, impeding the possible medicinal development of the drug.

3. Interest is Reviving in the Twenty-First Century:

- A resurgence of interest in psychedelic research occurred in the early 2000s, driven by developments in neuroscience and a more sophisticated comprehension of mental health.

- Pioneering experiments, like those carried out by scientists at Johns Hopkins University, reignited interest in psilocybin's medicinal potential among scientists.

4. Novel Research and Clinical Experiments:

- Over the past ten years, psilocybin's effects on mental health have been the subject of an unprecedented number of thorough clinical research.

- Research has been conducted on a variety of illnesses, such as PTSD, anxiety, and depression. Some of these studies have shown encouraging outcomes in terms of symptom relief and enhanced wellbeing.

5. Acceptance and Integration with the Mainstream:

• There has been a noticeable change in the scientific and medical professions' views regarding psychedelics in recent years.

• Continuous efforts are being made to include psilocybin into the mainstream of mental health care, since it is becoming more and more acknowledged as a viable therapy choice.

6. International Acknowledgment and Policy Assessment:

• Due to increased awareness of psilocybin's therapeutic potential, legislative changes and reevaluations of the drug's legal status in some jurisdictions have occurred on a global scale.

Research on the medicinal effects of psilocybin has developed over time, reflecting the dynamic interaction of scientific advancement, societal perceptions, and legal regulations. Ongoing research promises to provide further understanding of the workings and possible uses of this fascinating psychedelic substance

in mental health treatment as the
area develops.

Chapter Three

Magic mushroom usage in traditional cultures

Magic mushrooms, or mushrooms that contain the hallucinogenic ingredient psilocybin, have long been used in a variety of civilizations and geographical areas worldwide. These archaic customs offer insightful information on the cultural, spiritual, and historical significance of these fungi. Here are some instances of how magic mushrooms have been used traditionally:

1. American Indian and Native American Cultures

• Indigenous peoples throughout Mesoamerica, especially the Aztecs and the Mazatec people of Mexico, have traditionally used psilocybin-containing mushrooms.

• Psilocybin mushrooms were utilized in religious ceremonies and were known by the Aztecs as "teonanácatl," or "flesh of the gods." The belief behind this term was that it allowed for communion with deities.

2. Shamanism of the Mazatecs:

• The ceremonial usage of psilocybin mushrooms is part of a rich legacy of shamanic rituals among the Mazatec people

• Renowned Mazatec curandera (healer) Maria Sabina became well-known around the world for her work educating Westerners about the ceremonial usage of psilocybin mushrooms.

3. Indian Customs in Central and South America:

• The Shipibo-Conibo people of the Amazon rainforest, among other indigenous cultures in

Central and South America, have included psilocybin-containing mushrooms in their healing and spiritual practices.

• Using these mushrooms is frequently linked to healing, spiritual guidance, and insight-gathering.

4. African Traditional Medicine:

• Traditionally, certain African civilizations have used local psychotropic plants and fungi, such as mushrooms, in healing rituals.

• Though the methods differ throughout tribes and areas,

mushrooms are occasionally used as divination or ancestor spirit communication instruments.

5. Witchcraft in Historical Europe:

• Historical references imply that the usage of hallucinogenic mushrooms, such as flying ointments thought to contain ingredients like Amanita muscaria, may have been a part of some European witchcraft traditions.

6. Current Indigenous Methods:

• In certain areas, native groups continue to have cultural and spiritual ties to magic mushrooms, and they continue to use the plants in traditional ways.

Chapter Four

How psilocybin is converted by the body to psilocin

Psilocybin is a naturally occurring hallucinogenic substance that can be found in magic mushrooms, which are certain species of mushrooms. Following ingestion, psilocybin is transformed by the body's metabolic process into psilocin, the active substance that causes the euphoric effects. Here is how the procedure is broken down:

1. Chemical Composition:

• Psilocybin is a prodrug of psilocin; the two have similar structural makeup's. An inert substance that, when administered, becomes an active drug is known as a prodrug.

2. Consumption:

● Psilocybin-containing magic mushrooms are usually consumed orally, either by eating the mushrooms whole or steeping them in tea.

3. Take-up:

• Psilocybin is absorbed by the gastrointestinal tract after consumption of the mushrooms. Although it starts in the stomach, the small intestine is where the majority of the process happens.

4 Psilocin Conversion:

• Psilocin is produced when the enzyme alkaline phosphatase breaks down psilocybin. This enzyme converts psilocybin into psilocin by removing the phosphate group.

5.Transport of Blood:

• The bloodstream then quickly absorbs psilocin and carries it to the brain. Psilocin is able to pass past the blood-brain barrier thanks to this process that takes place in the circulatory system.

6. Serotonin Receptor Interaction:

- Psilocin mostly interacts with serotonin receptors in the brain, specifically the 5-HT2A receptor. Because of their structural resemblance, psilocin and serotonin can bind to these receptors and influence serotoninergic neurotransmission.

7. Impact on the Nervous System:

- Psilocin activates serotonin receptors, which modifies neuronal firing patterns and neurotransmitter release. The typical psychedelic effects, such as altered perception, mood, and cognitive function, are the outcome of this modulation.

8. Effects Duration:

• Depending on the dosage and individual circumstances, the effects of psilocin usually reach their peak one to two hours after consumption and can continue for several hours.

9. Removal:

• The liver finally breaks down psilocin, which the body then excretes as urine.

Serotonin receptor interaction and its effects on brain function

The hallucinogenic effects of magic mushrooms are primarily caused by the interaction of psilocin, the active metabolite of psilocybin, with serotonin receptors. The following summarizes the effects of psilocin on brain function and how it interacts with serotonin receptors:

1. Binding to Receptors for Serotonin:

• Serotonin, a neurotransmitter involved in mood regulation and other physiological activities, and psilocin share structural similarities. Serotonin receptors, particularly the 5-HT2A receptor subtype, are the primary target of psilocin's binding.

2. Control of Serotonin Transmission Modulation:

• Psilocin modifies serotoninergic neurotransmission by binding to serotonin receptors. It throws off the regular cycles of serotonin release and absorption.

3. Enhanced Release of Serotonin:

• In some areas of the brain, psilocin promotes the release of serotonin. This rise in serotonin levels is part of the overall change in the brain's neurotransmitter balance.

4. Improved Neural Networks:

• Psilocin stimulates serotonin receptors, which increases brain connection. Changes in perception, emotion, and cognitive patterns are among the psychedelic effects that may be caused by this enhanced communication across brain regions.

5. Modified Activity on the Default Mode Network (DMN):

• It has been demonstrated that psilocin reduces activity in the brain network known as the default mode, which is connected to self-referential thought and ego. This modification could play a role in the breakdown of barriers that occur between the psychedelic experience and the outside world.

6. Effect on Emotion and Mood:

• Changes in mood and emotion are associated with psilocin's regulation of serotonin receptors. Increased empathy, heightened emotional experiences, and a sense of oneness are frequently reported by users.

7. Effects on cognition:

- Psilocin can alter perception, creativity, and cognition through its interaction with serotonin receptors. It's possible for users to develop new cognitive patterns and improved introspection.

8. Neuroplasticity and Its Potential for Therapy:

- According to some research, psilocin's psychedelic experience may encourage neuroplasticity, which could be a factor in the drug's therapeutic effects. This is especially important when discussing mental health issues like PTSD, anxiety, and despair.

It's important to remember that research is still being done to determine the exact processes and total influence of psilocin on brain function. A key component of the psychedelic experience is the interaction with serotonin receptors, which may help us comprehend the possible benefits and hazards of using magic mushrooms.

Chapter Five

Important discoveries made during clinical trials regarding mental health issues

The key ingredient in magic mushrooms, psilocybin, has showed encouraging results in clinical trials investigating its therapeutic potential for treating a range of mental health issues. Here are some significant discoveries from clinical trials, but research is still ongoing:

1. Depression

• Psilocybin-assisted therapy has been shown in clinical trials to significantly reduce depression symptoms. Research, like those done at Johns Hopkins University and Imperial College London, has shown that individuals with treatment-resistant depression experience long-lasting benefits and an overall improvement in their well-being.

2. Disorders of Anxiety:

• In patients with life-threatening conditions, psilocybin has demonstrated promise in reducing symptoms of anxiety disorders, such as existential anguish and generalized anxiety. Studies have shown that when paired with psychological support, a single psilocybin dosage can produce long-lasting anxiety reductions.

3. PTSD, or post-traumatic stress disorder:

● Psilocybin's potential as a PTSD treatment has been investigated in a few clinical studies. According to preliminary research, psilocybin-assisted treatment may lessen symptoms of post-traumatic stress disorder and assist people in processing traumatic experiences. However, more investigation is required to confirm its safety and effectiveness in wider populations.

4. Treatment for Addiction:

• Psilocybin's potential to treat substance use disorders, such as addiction to alcohol and tobacco, has been studied. Psilocybin-assisted treatment has been linked in studies to better mood and higher rates of abstinence, which may help break addictive habits.

5. Terminal Illness and Existential Distress:

• Psilocybin has been studied in clinical studies for patients with life-threatening conditions including cancer in an effort to reduce existential anguish and enhance quality of life. The findings suggest that a single psilocybin dose given in a therapeutically encouraging environment can result in significant and long-lasting improvements in attitude and perspective toward life and death.

6. Connectivity and Neuroplasticity:

• Studies using imaging techniques both during and after psilocybin sessions have shown alterations in brain connection and activity. The default mode network (DMN) appears to be altered by psilocybin, which may contribute to its therapeutic benefits by increasing neuronal connection and possibly causing neuroplastic changes.

The area of psychedelic-assisted therapy is still in its infancy, so even while these results are encouraging, additional study is required to determine the safety, effectiveness, and long-term effects of psilocybin in many mental health contexts. Furthermore, these therapies are usually administered in environments under the guidance and supervision of qualified specialists.

Depression

Promising findings have been found in the research on psilocybin's therapeutic potential for depression, especially when it comes to treatment-resistant depression. The following are important discoveries of psilocybin and depression:

1. Diminished Indications of Depression:

● Research from clinical studies has demonstrated that psilocybin can significantly and quickly reduce depressed symptoms when taken as a single dose in a supportive and regulated environment. Improvements in outlook, general well-being, and mood are frequently reported by participants.

2. Long-Term Impacts:

•   Research has shown that psilocybin's antidepressant effects can last for a long time. Following just one psilocybin session, participants in certain trials have experienced continuing gains for weeks or even months.

3. Changes in Neuroplasticity and Connectivity:

•   Neuronal connection has changed in the brain during and after psilocybin sessions, according to imaging studies. The default mode network (DMN), a brain network linked to self-referential thought, appears to be impacted by psilocybin. Modifications in dopaminergic neuron activity are associated with antidepressant effects and may signify enhanced neuroplasticity.

4. Integration of Psychotherapy:

• Psychotherapeutic integration is a common component of psilocybin-assisted treatment, in which patients reflect and have conversations with their therapists in order to incorporate new perspectives from their psychedelic experience into their everyday lives. It is believed that this integration process adds to the therapeutic advantages.

5. Effectiveness in Depression Refractory to Treatment:

• People with treatment-resistant depression, a difficult condition that does not respond well to traditional antidepressant drugs, have demonstrated success with psilocybin. Psilocybin's unique methods of action might provide a fresh strategy for people who have not responded to conventional therapies.

6. Tolerance and Safety:

• Studies indicate that psilocybin is generally well tolerated when used under strict guidelines and after proper screening. The acute psychedelic effects are transient, and serious adverse reactions are uncommon.

7. Attitude and Context:

• The state of mind and environment in which an experience takes place affect psilocybin's therapeutic benefits. Research highlights how crucial it is to have a safe, well-planned atmosphere in order to maximize the benefits of psilocybin-assisted therapy.

8. Current Research and Upcoming Paths:

- Psilocybin and depression research is a rapidly developing field. The goals of ongoing study are to better understand the mechanisms of action, enhance treatment regimens, and investigate the possibility of incorporating psilocybin into conventional mental health services.

Chapter Six

Summary of research on depression diseases

A review of research using psilocybin to treat depression disorders sheds light on how psychedelic-assisted therapy is developing. Key elements and conclusions from numerous investigations are as follows:

1. Cutting-Edge Research:

• Early research on psychedelics in the 2000s, carried out by scientists like Roland Griffiths at Johns Hopkins University, was crucial in reviving interest in the field. The groundwork for investigating psilocybin's effects on consciousness and mood was established by these investigations.

2. Studies at Johns Hopkins University:

• Studies carried out at Johns Hopkins University have been crucial in proving that psilocybin may have therapeutic benefits for depression disorders. Research indicates that when paired with psychological assistance, a single psilocybin dosage can result in notable decreases in depressed symptoms.

3. Research from Imperial College London:

● Research conducted at Imperial College London, particularly work by Robin Carhart-Harris, has advanced our knowledge of the brain mechanisms underpinning psilocybin's antidepressant benefits. Changes in brain connection patterns have been found in imaging studies, especially in the default mode network (DMN), which is linked to self-referential thought.

4. Trial by Usona Institute, Phase 2:

● A Phase 2 clinical trial was carried out by the Usona Institute to examine the safety and effectiveness of psilocybin for major depressive disorder (MDD). According to preliminary data, participants' depressed symptoms significantly improved. These results are encouraging.

5. Research Funded by MAPS:

The use of psilocybin and other psychedelics for a variety of mental health disorders, including depression, has been the subject of research supported by the Multidisciplinary Association for Psychedelic Studies (MAPS). Their research emphasizes the value of a supportive therapy environment while concentrating on strict techniques.

6. Depression Resistant to Treatment:

• Treatment-resistant depression, a disorder in which people do not react well to standard antidepressant drugs, has been the focus of several investigations. Psilocybin has demonstrated effectiveness in alleviating symptoms for those suffering from this difficult type of depression.

7. Integration of Psychotherapy:

• A lot of research highlights the value of psychotherapy integration, in which patients discuss their experiences and incorporate new understandings into their daily life with licensed therapists. It is thought that this integration process is essential to the long-term therapeutic benefits of psilocybin.

8. Safety and Moral Issues Must Be Considered

• Safety and ethical issues are also emphasized in investigations on psilocybin and depressive illnesses. Studies are carried out in controlled settings to reduce dangers, and participant suitability is ensured by the use of screening procedures.

9. Current and Upcoming Studies:

• Research into the mechanisms of action of psilocybin, treatment protocols, and its possible integration into standard mental health care are all ongoing and planned projects in this dynamic sector.

Even if the results are encouraging, it's important to interpret them cautiously and recognize that more investigation, extensive clinical studies, and long-term follow-ups are required to determine the safety and effectiveness of psilocybin in treating depressive disorders.

Success stories and difficulties in using psilocybin to cure depression

Success Narratives:

1. Considerable Mitigation of Symptoms:

• Many patients undergoing psilocybin-assisted depression therapy report notable improvements in their depressive symptoms. These success tales frequently involve feelings of emotional alleviation, general well-being, and mood enhancements.

2.Long-Term Advantages:

- Psilocybin therapy has been shown to have long-lasting effects in certain success stories, where patients report continuing improvements in their mood and mental health weeks or months after just one session. This is not the case with traditional antidepressants, which may need to be taken every day.

3. Good Life Shifts:

- Success tales frequently include positive life improvements in addition to symptom relief.

Increased motivation, improved interpersonal connections, and a stronger sense of direction and meaning in life are possible outcomes reported by participants.

4. Enhanced Life Quality:

• Improvements in general quality of life are a common feature of psilocybin therapy success stories. Individuals may talk about a change in outlook, heightened resilience, and an improved capacity to deal with obstacles in life more skillfully.

5. Breaking the Rumination Cycle:

- It is sometimes said that psilocybin-assisted therapy breaks the habit of negative thinking and rumination that is connected to depression. Participants report experiencing a mental shift that has improved their clarity and optimism when facing obstacles

Problems:

1. Absence of Standardization

- The absence of established treatment guidelines presents a difficulty when using psilocybin to treat depression, It can be difficult to build a consistent strategy because different studies and clinical settings may use different dosage, session structures, and integration procedures.

2. Legal and Moral Obstacles:

• Because psilocybin is categorized as a Schedule I controlled substance in many jurisdictions, research and clinical use may face regulatory obstacles. Careful thought must also be given to ethical issues pertaining to participant safety and wellbeing.

3. Personal Differences:

Individuals' reactions to psilocybin therapy differ greatly. While some people have significant and beneficial results, others might not react favorably or might even experience negative side effects. One major challenge is to understand and anticipate individual variability.

4. Restricted Durational Information:

• There are few long-term studies on the effectiveness and safety of psilocybin for depression. More thorough research is required to evaluate the long-term effects and potential hazards of continuous use, as most trials have rather short follow-up periods.

5. Assistance with Integration:

• Maintaining positive results requires a successful integration of the psychedelic experience into daily life. If people don't have the resources and help to integrate the insights they acquired from the psychedelic session, problems could occur.

6. The public's perception and stigma:

• Psilocybin's legitimacy as a depression treatment may be

hampered by the stigma attached to psychedelics and a lack of public understanding. Overcoming false information and societal stereotypes is a constant struggle.

Uncertainty

Psilocybin therapy for anxiety has been studied, and the findings are encouraging, especially for disorders like existential anxiety and generalized anxiety disorder (GAD). The following summarizes the main research results on psilocybin and anxiety:

1. Diminished Anxiety Symptoms:

● Clinical investigations have shown that psilocybin can lessen anxiety symptoms. A reduction in overall anxiety, which includes sensations of tension, restlessness, and apprehension, is frequently reported by participants.

2. Cancer Patients' Existential Anxiety:

Research has concentrated on reducing existential anxiety in patients with cancer and other life-threatening conditions. The use of psilocybin in conjunction with treatment has demonstrated potential in facilitating deep spiritual and existential experiences, which can lessen anxiety associated with dread of dying.

3. Enhanced Release of Emotions:

• It has been observed that psilocybin increases the release of emotions during therapeutic sessions. This emotional catharsis can aid in the healing process by enabling people to face and address the underlying problems that are causing their anxiety.

## 4.	Improved	Emotional Intelligence

• Psilocybin's effects on serotonin receptors may improve the brain's ability to process emotions. This may make it easier to react more adaptably to stimuli and help lessen the sensations of anxiety.

5. Long-Term Advantages:

• According to certain research, psilocybin's beneficial benefits on anxiety may last long after the psychedelic experience. Individuals may have long-lasting reductions in anxiety and depression, which would improve their overall quality of life.

6. Traditional Medical Interventions vs. Psilocybin-Assisted Therapy:

- Studies comparing psilocybin-assisted therapy to traditional anxiety therapies such selective serotonin reuptake inhibitors (SSRIs) have been conducted. Some results suggest that psilocybin might offer deeper and quicker alleviation, but more studies are required to determine its relative effectiveness.

7. Changes in Neural Connectivity:

- Psilocybin alters brain connectivity, especially in areas linked to emotional processing, according to neuroimaging research. These changes could be part of the therapeutic benefits seen in anxiety disorders.

Chapter Seven

Things to Think About:

1. Safety Issues:

- Although psilocybin has demonstrated a largely positive safety profile in controlled environments, negative responses and psychological distress are possible. To reduce dangers, careful screening and supervision are necessary.

2. Personal Differences:

- There can be significant individual variation in psilocybin responses. The type and strength of a psychedelic experience can vary depending on a number of factors, including personality, past experiences, and mental health history.

3. A Legal and Ethical Perspective:

• Many jurisdictions regard psilocybin to be a controlled substance, and using it in therapeutic contexts presents moral and legal questions. The morality of using psilocybin-assisted therapy and its accessibility are topics of continuous discussion.

4. Assistance with Integration

• For long-lasting therapeutic advantages, integrating the

psychedelic experience into daily life is essential. Having enough resources and support for integration is crucial to a thorough treatment plan.

In order to potentially include psilocybin into standard mental health care, it will be imperative to address these issues and get a deeper grasp of the subtleties of its therapeutic mechanisms as research on the drug and anxiety progresses.

Investigating the effects of psilocybin on anxiety disorders

Recent years have seen a major increase in the amount of

research on the effects of psilocybin on anxiety disorders, with an increasing number of studies pointing to possible therapeutic advantages. The following examines some of the main points of psilocybin and anxiety disorders:

1. Diminution of All-Over Anxiety:

• Psilocybin may help to lessen generalized anxiety, according to studies and clinical trials. After having psychedelic experiences, participants frequently report feeling calmer and experiencing less overall anxiety.

2. End-of-Life Distress and Existential Anxiety:

• Treatment with psilocybin has demonstrated potential in reducing existential anxiety, particularly in patients with serious diseases. Particularly those suffering from cancer have reported significant psychological and emotional relief, which has enhanced their quality of life and lessened their suffering as they approach death.

3. Quick Relief onset:

• One noteworthy aspect noted in certain research is how quickly anxiety symptoms can be relieved following a single psilocybin session. In comparison, conventional psychiatric drugs can take weeks to produce noticeable results.

4. Improved Emotional Intelligence

• It is believed that psilocybin improves emotional processing, enabling people to face and deal with repressed feelings that might be linked to anxiety disorders. Those who engage in psychedelic experiences may have a rare chance to learn more about their emotional terrain.

5. Brain Connectivity and Neuroplasticity:

• Studies using neuroimaging have demonstrated that psilocybin alters the patterns of brain connectivity. Changes to the default mode network (DMN), a part of the brain linked to self-referential thought, are among them. The therapeutic benefits seen in anxiety disorders could be attributed in part to these modifications.

6. Anxiety That Resists Treatment:

• When it comes to people with anxiety problems who have not responded to standard therapies, psilocybin has showed promise. Psilocybin's unique mechanisms of action might provide an alternate strategy for people who have not responded to conventional therapies.

Obstacles & Things to Think About:

1. Security and Guidance:

- The security of patients receiving psilocybin-assisted therapy is of utmost importance. To reduce risks and bad responses, appropriate screening, preparation, and therapy supervision are crucial.

2. Personal Differences:

● There can be significant individual variation in psilocybin responses. The results of the psychedelic experience can be influenced by variables like personality, anxiety disorder kind, and psychiatric history.

3. A Legal and Ethical Perspective:

● Psilocybin's legal position and ethical administration in therapeutic settings continue to be problematic issues. Achieving an appropriate incorporation of psilocybin into mental health care requires navigating these considerations.

4.   Assistance   with Integration:

• For long-lasting therapeutic effects, integration support—discussions with licensed therapists to assist clients in processing and integrating newfound insights—is essential.

The ethical development and implementation of psilocybin-assisted therapy in the context of anxiety disorders will depend on resolving these issues and developing a thorough grasp of the drug's therapeutic potential as research on psilocybin and anxiety disorders advances.